# LET THERE BE WELLNESS
## Don't Block It!
### By
### ETTA DIXON

Published in the United States by House of Walker
Publishing, LLC (HWP) New Jersey

Permissions:
Copyright © 2025 by Etta Dixon
Let There be Wellness (Don't Block It!)
ISBN: 978-1-957775-05-0
LCCN: 2025917480

\* Nothing in this book should be considered medical advice.
All dietary suggestions should be discussed with your
medical provider before implementation.

# Miss Etta Dixon

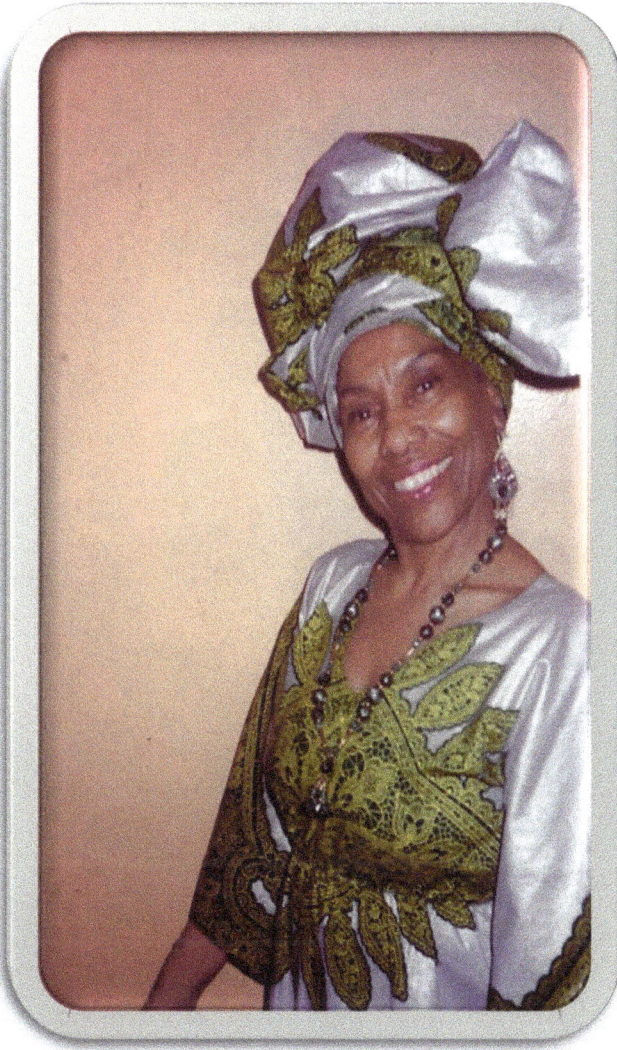

It is my joy to welcome you to read my book. I want you to receive this joy. We both will be satisfied!

I take great pleasure to remind all of you of an important heritage we received from our great grandparents. It was not land nor money, and it wasn't property. It was something more valuable than all three above. It was the thing they used to heal the sick. It always worked. That thing was fresh grown herbs and vegetables. No doctor prescriptions for them. They didn't go to doctors. They had a choice of more than three thousand vegetables and herbs. I thank the past generations for this information, and I promise to continue to pass it on to future generations. Hear ye Hear ye! Eating fresh grown vegetables and herbs will never block your wellness. Try it!

# TABLE OF CONTENTS

# PREFACE

*'Let There be Wellness (Don't Block It!)'* is an excellent book, chock full of healing information. I am also the author of *'I'm a Wellness Witness,'* written with you in mind. Both books are powerful guides to develop your portrait of wellness. My books reveal how every part of your anatomy needs the energy of healthy organs and very good circulation in order to obtain a satisfactory bill of good health. This knowledge prepares you for the necessary adjustments that will not only swing you into good health but will produce trend seekers who want a piece of the wellness pie.

Before you embark on your portrait of wellness, I need to prepare you so that it can be a delightful transition. Right now, I'm sure you have a small wellness routine, but a heartfelt, healthy, book reading, should broaden your quest for complete healing.

From this day, hour, and minute, please clear your mind from disease and negative thinking. Such clutter can be a turnoff for any pleasant, healthy thoughts to enter the brain. Remember, my main prescription (from my first book, *'I'm a Wellness Witness,'* is: TRAIN BRAIN! IN DEALING WITH HEALING, PREVENTION IS THE INTENTION!

When a doctor diagnoses a patient with high blood pressure, high blood sugar and high cholesterol, this immediately elicits a decline in his/her self-esteem and self-worth. This diagnosis transmits a sick report, although there was no sick feeling before examination. Now is the time for the light bulb to come on letting you know that you can completely heal. Let your strength come through and ask the question, *what can I do to completely heal?* This is the main reason I write books. There's no time to feel sorry for yourself. Instead, use every minute of your future to heal your body.

When you are stricken by a doctor's unhealthy report, what do you do? The first thing you should do is to PAY ATTENTION to what your body is saying! Most of us have a habit of ignoring our body language and other symptoms. We also have a habit of buying over-the-counter remedies, forgetting about the non-medicated remedies our parents and grandparents successfully used. Prepare to investigate the situation thoroughly. Instead of jumping the gun to use new things, make an effort to hear an elder's herbal story.

This book is written purposely to give a deeper insight into unfamiliar predicaments, and to encourage you to pay close attention to what your body is saying to you. For instance, pain, or a fever, are rock-solid signs that possibly a serious illness is coming. This book offers words of encouragement and wisdom from an elder who has been ill only once in her entire life. Although preventative information is limited, we can still train ourselves early in life to be a health detective. Engaging in preventive care can be a welcome way to get the disease dilemma to disappear, preventing sickness from festering before awful damage appears.

We, (you and I), can offer ordinary measures of how to handle subtle misfortunes. Denial is unacceptable. For example, pain is a warning; you should: 1. Try to ascertain why there's pain 2. See your provider and 3. Eat healthier vegetables and fruits.

Be aware that healing early is easier. Healing early is tranquil care vs trauma care. We want to embrace wellness before the trauma sets in. Let There Be Wellness, Hurry! Don't Block It! Let the following be the catalyst to wellness.

# ORDERS

• Make self-care, your self-care, a habit

• Welcome what helps you, avoid what harms you.

• MEND - Place yourself in a healing environment.

• Your body is a spiritual link to GOD. Healing demands a positive state of mind.

• Squeeze your leg muscles a few times. It'll help your blood jump to the heart (I do this often and have never had a heart attack). This improves your circulation because it gets the blood back to your heart.

The wellness message chapters can be a therapeutic journey for all. Knowing what you must work on is a huge help. You know the things you do right. You know the wrong things you do. Put yourself on a mission, make this decision--right things you keep and wrong things you wean off. The first law of nature is self-preservation. Get on the road to health rejuvenation. Become your own personal trainer and do everything that helps you. Do nothing that hurts you.

## STRAIGHT FORWARD MESSAGE STRATEGY

• Always emphasize tranquil care (it takes needed transition time).

• Think miracle wellness. I experienced it.

• Embrace family wellness immediately.

• Slow down pursuing matrimony and look to elders for clear input. Matrimony now may be too soon. Save yourself.

• Allow lots of wisdom to enter your life as soon as possible.

• Pursue financial wellness. I serve as an example in my financial journey documented in this book.

• Practice educational wellness. Never lack knowledge.

- Dance. Women especially enjoy this. It's therapeutic wellness.
- Grasp spiritual wellness. It's a jewel to behold.
- Keep your brain alert. Engage in everything.
- Polish your wellness knowledge.
- This list is a jewel for happiness.

Portraits of wellness serves as another heartfelt journey for me. My writings have helped me recognize a certain focal point from my Creator. It is the concept of the age expectancy the Creator has perpetrated for His creation. *'Let There Be Wellness'* is a map to ensure the path of a centurion with GOD's help and barring accidents. We were designed to live to one hundred years of age without Alzheimer's or any other disorder. All we need is to do follow the natural protocol of wellness.

I have truly been blessed to reach 92 years of age with no aches or pains, and I have reason to believe that I am on target to see one hundred. I give thanks for His gifts of air, water, stars, sun, moon, trees, grass, flowers and colors. We were created to enjoy life and be happy. I want to satisfy this aspiration of God and hopefully you do too.

Let *'Let There Be Wellness Don't block It,'* be your guide in fulfilling a long happy healthier life. Becoming a member of the 100 plus club is doable. If one is in tuned to self and recognize that some of your cells rejuvenate every seven years. We just have to be sure that we don't go over our quota of body toxins and poisons. The way we can do this is to remember: the berry is your food, the herbs are your medicine, and the animals are your pets. Eating this way allows the body to refurbish in a healthy manner every 7 years. Eating fresh fruits and vegetables accelerates the body's wellness.

# DEDICATION

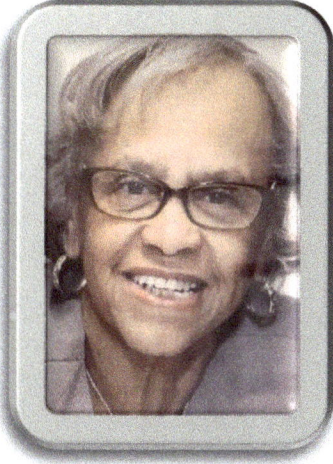

This book is dedicated to Mrs. Wilnette Jones with tons of love, warm feelings and happiness. Wilnette is the example to follow when you desire to achieve family dedication. Her first step began by becoming a devoted wife. Wilnette is the widow of Mr. Jerome W. Jones, Sr., and the mother of Artist Jeromyah W. Jones (whom I'd like to introduce). Next, she worked on quiet, smooth, family wellness.

Artist Jeromyah W. Jones' wife of 43 years, Kemery Jones, is a great fit into the Jones' family record of devotion. They have an adult son named Jeromyah, who throughout his lifetime, maintained the information on the Black freedom leaders that his father compiled. Jeromyah made a tremendous contribution to the freedom movement with his printout of 75 Black human rights leaders (printout below). These leaders paved the way to freedom. He made history in creating this printout of which, should be in every school. It would be a revelation for students. Many of them know very few Black civil rights leaders and are starving for this information. Using this, we can enlighten future generations to continue the work. They achieved it, now, like Jeromyah, we need to do our part to maintain it. (You can also check out Jeromyah's website for more information:

(wwwjeromewjonesjr.com)

Jeromyah is also aware of the work that still needs to be done. Thank God for the Jones family. We must not lose what they worked so hard to achieve. We are responsible for honoring our descendants and keeping their stories alive.

# INTRODUCTION

This book, *'Let there be Wellness (Don't Block It!),* gives a direct path to healthy living. It is done through helpmates, and they are as follows:

1.  Elder Asantewaa Gale Harris
Community Vision Council 646-544-1095
Referrals - Such as grass roots and a collection of farmers markets.
2.Outreach of speakers and health fairs
Toolkits for Healthy Choices & Healthy Living.

She is also responsible for my connection to King Spa, which I have been attending most Wednesdays starting from 2007. (I attended the 10th St. bathhouse for twenty years).

2. Felicia Watkis 718-469-7262
Felicia prepares delicious raw salads and transitional food that will get you to the raw food.

She also knows a lot of helpful wellness tips. She is a master chef. Her natural food preparation never hurt anyone.

3. Lola Rozier

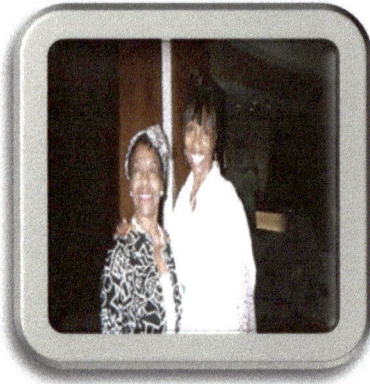

She advocated for Juneteenth to become a recognized holiday. Her efforts, along with the efforts of many others, succeeded in this endeavor. Sometimes, it takes many people to help you reach your wellness goals and she is one of the people who helped me. Others may be medical professionals, healthy family members, or a health advisor. I want you to call this the Disease Prevention Wellness Extension Connection: Reach out to their organization at 718-469-7262. Leave a message and someone will get back to you.

## BLACK (FREEDOM HUMAN RIGHTS LEADERS

I want to make this important introduction of Black (Freedom} Human Rights Leaders. The following printout is by my artistic cousin, Jerome Jones Sr.

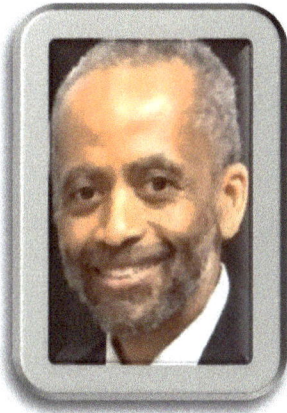

Once I received a copy of the printout, the thought came to me to present them in my book. The idea hit me when I heard a teenage boy say to us something that I never thought I would ever hear from a teenager. It was the hurt I felt, and saw in him, when he presented the following question:

*"Why didn't somebody tell me that there was a man named Malcom X walking the streets of Harlem and talking to the Black people about racism."*

*"Do we have a democracy or a hypocrisy"*? Malcome X asked. It is a great question. Each of his speeches were more stimulating than the last, and his fame skyrocketed. He even traveled to the motherland and fought for human rights.

After hearing this teenager's simple cry, I decided that artist Jeromyah Jones Jr.'s printout of 1978 will no longer be a secret. Now, you will find the printout here. I have included twenty faces and names of these leaders to share with the world (the remaining will be in my next book *'Let There Be Wellness, Stop supporting Sickness.'*

On the following page, you will see faces of Black men and women who had so much wellness in them, that they paved the way to freedom for us followers. Strong, Black, healthy people who were healthy enough to do it, left a road map for us to continue our fight for freedom. We thank all of these good people. Choose one to follow with ease and he or she will be incredibly grateful. They provided the way for us to go, and go we shall, because we are well.

Many generations after Malcom's death, those who knew nothing of Malcom's outstanding work in civil rights, need to learn the news about others who paved the way for our civil rights. This unique printout can be helpful in opening the eyes of our youth about what went on before they were born. The sooner they learn about Black history, the better. It will enhance their decision-making power in life. This is an important quality we need to quickly grasp and work on.

Ingenious

African Minds by

Jerome W. Jones

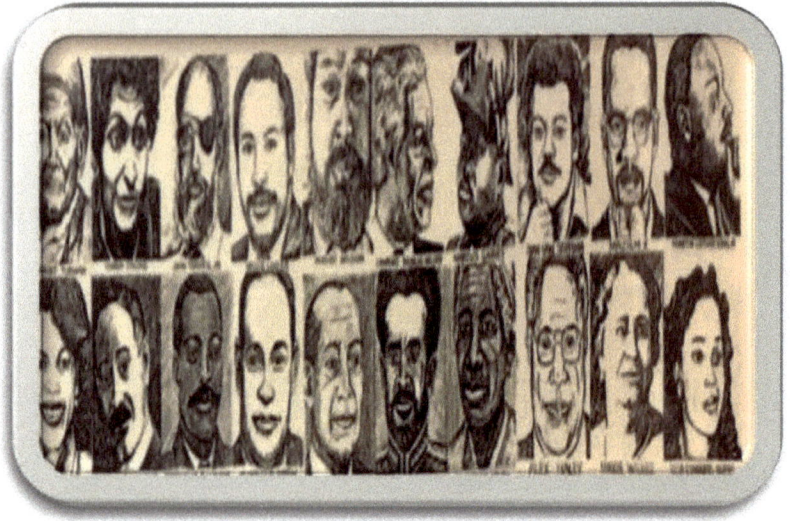

Choose one leader from the following printout and decide to continue his/her work. Ask a friend to join you. It will be a nice, brain strengthening experience for both of you. Enjoy your newfound adventure. Don't forget to drop a note on Amazon reviews. I need the feedback.

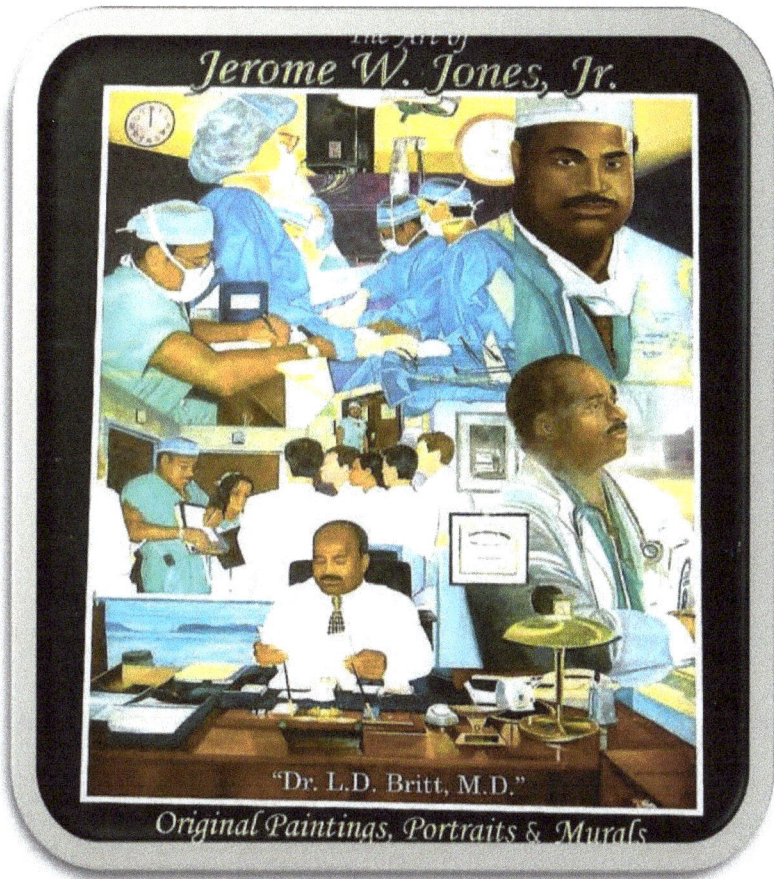

The Art of
*Jerome W. Jones, Jr.*

"Dr. L.D. Britt, M.D."

*Original Paintings, Portraits & Murals*

**FREEDOM…You MUST read BLACK IS THE COLOR by Ruth Duckett Gibbs**

We Need Yesterday's Leaders Today! Bring them back inside of you and continue their work: Harriet Tubman, ML King Jr., Rosa Parks, Malcolm X. The list continues in this book.

Vigor and vitality, the desired energy for success. We live in a capitalistic system. Why not capitalize on capitalism? I mean the positive way. Then, we all can get benefits. Our civil rights leaders taught us the way to use our wits by learning how to follow – POSITIVITY. It shouldn't be a missing factor. Leaders exude extra vitality, hoping to interest youth in customizing their dynamism and continuing what our civil rights leaders started.

Back in my day, people ate organic food. It was grown locally and cooked at home. We weighed in the hundreds, never six hundred. What crossed the lips was fresh nourishment, anything else was deemed unacceptable. Human right leaders did the things they knew directed them to victory – what is stopping us– open your eyes wide, see leaders paving the way. Believe me, it is doable for us and we can deliver. It will please me if you pick one leader and continue what he/she started.

# Miracle Wellness

Approximately four years before my surgery, on a Monday, in the month of October of 1933, I, Etta Chase (aka 'May'), was born. I was named after my mother. It was a time when the famous Depression was at its lowest slump. Millionaires committed suicide and unemployed citizens became apple vendors. This crisis was always remembered by my mother. She often said, *"I had to stand on a soup line in order to eat."*

I was born into a poor family of four which consisted of my maternal grandparents, Nathaniel Clark and Mattie Clark, my mama Etta Chase, and my sister Margaret. Margaret was three years my senior. She was no easy act to follow. She was such a good baby. She hardly cried and slept a great deal of the time. She was a perfect baby as far as Ma was concerned. She made sure that no one forgot it but she did worry about her when she had the whooping cough. I, on the other hand, wound up in the hospital with a deadly medical emergency.

*"Please doctor,"* said Etta Chase to the doctor at Cumberland Hospital's emergency room, *"Tell me. Why is my baby crying day and night?"* My mother couldn't take any more of my frenzied cries. She finally decided to take me to the emergency room (in the early 20th century it was a luxury for poor families to go to a hospital). *"I don't know,"* said the doctor. *"Let me examine your child."* With these words, the doctor pressed down on my lower stomach area, causing me to holler louder than ever before. Ignoring my cries, the doctor proceeded to press even harder on the side of my stomach. Now I released a sound that was twice as shrilled and piercing. At the same time, I kicked the doctor. My mother was stunned, mortified. What kind of monster was causing this type of reaction from her baby?

After ex-rays were taken, the doctors learned that my appendix erupted. Peritonitis had taken over my small body. In the nineteen-thirties, this disease caused full-grown adults to meet their maker. How could a tiny baby survive with a body full of poison? Emergency surgery was set up immediately. Although mother was told that there was no hope, they still did the operation (this was a way for student doctors to get experience, maybe that was why they operated).

The tedious process of removing venom from a toddler's blood was accomplished through cutting into the ankle and placing a drainage tube that allowed the contaminated blood to drain out (it was the only safe area to do blood work on a very small child). Inserting tube allowed fresh blood to enter my waning body. My entire bloodline was changed, and my entire stomach was cut in order to remove my ruptured appendix. Not only was the surgery a success, I, the patient, lived, and family, friends and doctors, got a happy shock. Later, no doctor believed it was one appendix and one surgery. As I grew, the cuts on my stomach grew apart and a different doctor would ask, *"What was these surgeries for?"* They didn't believe me when I told them it was just one surgery. Today, it looks like one small incision. The slashing wounds where the transfer of blood was made on my ankle, are still visible today.

After I was pieced back together with countless stitches, my endless crying returned. This time, it was a little simpler. I was sent to a convalescence home for three months. This was to ensure my recovery. Since I was a child of four years or less, I cried for my mother. I wanted her that minute, not three months later. I felt that my hospital stay was more than enough absenteeism between her and I. An orphan child never felt lonelier than I did at that moment. I just couldn't stop crying. The attendants at the convalescence home engaged the help of

Mother Nature. They said, *"Let's put her outside in the garden."* I stopped crying immediately because in my mind, being outside was getting me closer to my ma.

At last, the three months (of prison) were over and I joyfully returned home to face another scenario. Suddenly, the nightmare my family had just gone through became the daily, if not hourly, topic discussed with the neighbors. No listener escaped. It was extra news, hear all about it. Ma vented to as many listeners as possible about how our family miracle was almost a family tragedy. The climax of the story was when a viewing of my hacked stomach was uncovered. They had never seen any surgery like it; the horror was displayed on their faces. It was a most traumatizing experience for a person at such a young age. Even today, I remember the screaming cries I made at the top of my lungs for ma. I desperately wanted her consolation. I was most grateful that the doctor's prognosis was wrong when he said that I wouldn't survive. Well, survive I did and I made my first silent vow to live a life in pursuit of wellness (although I didn't know the vocabulary, I knew the desire).

My thanks were endless for my miracle wellness. This episode of sickness was so powerful it stirred me to welcome wellness forever. An experience so dramatic, it made my quest for a long healthy life, and it happened. I am 92 years young and the only surviving member of my immediate family. I give thanks for the operating doctor who returned me to life.

# Life after the miracle

I was quite a challenge to ma and that didn't include the surgery. She said that I was always fighting sleep. She didn't realize that my spot in the bed, which was barely equipped to sleep two, held me hostage between her and Margaret. Jammed between the two of them, I kept trying to find space to sleep. There wasn't any so I just spent the nights wide awake ensuring that I didn't get squashed. This earned my mother's description of me as always being fidgety. My movements always made her a nervous wreck. The coffee she drank was never to blame. She felt confident that it was me that kept her heart in her mouth. Also, she never forgot that it was I who bit her nipple when she was nursing me. Ma thought that I did it on purpose because I smiled afterwards but hungry me, was just trying to get the milk and when I got it, I was happy and held on tight.

I grew to be an energetic toddler, schoolgirl and teenager. My spirit was just too much for my mother. She even said she was going to examine me to see if I had ants in my pants. There was a whole list of things about me that seemed negative to my family. I always asked lots of questions. I really thought ma was my source for those answers, but she tried everything she could to put a halt to my high flow of questions and my extra energy. She really didn't know the answers to my questions and hated my always asking. After some time, I learned that the library was my best bet and started trailblazing there.

I was very shocked when in 1943, ma gave birth to Jacqueline. She never mentioned a word. She just came home from the hospital with her new baby. Nobody knew she was pregnant because she had an extended stomach anyway. With so many complaints about me, she still increased her family with a third daughter. My younger sister Jackie grew to join their way of thinking about me. Eventually, everyone was happy when they realized that Jackie was more like Margaret than me.

Life was slower then and they all surmised that I was too fast to last. I got used to it in my early years and took it in stride. In those days, children had to sit still and be quiet, especially girls (who were told to keep their dresses down).

My high energy got me into a lot of trouble. It also caused me to be a hearty eater. It caused me to wear out my clothes and shoes sooner than anyone else. This posed a serious burden on Ma who was in a financial deficit. Her job paid three dollars a week and she was separated from her husband whose income was probably less. She couldn't feed us, nor clothe us on a salary so low. In the forties, a Black woman's option for earning honest income was housework. She had to apply for welfare. They politely told her that she was ineligible because she had a father who had a secure job with the Pennsylvania Railroad as a porter. She was informed of the welfare policy: A working father was responsible for his daughter's children.

My gratitude is extended to Grandpa Nat for his care and financial provisions throughout my elementary, junior high and high school years. The foundation he gave me was genuinely welcomed. It contributed positively to my early wellness. I offer sincere thanks.

I also give thanks for my childhood because I certainly did not have to look for childhood after I grew up. I graciously accepted the early years even though, to me, they appeared to be extra-long. It was pretty easy to accept after all because we did not have TV, Nintendo, videos, VCRs, cell phones, internet, boom boxes or cable. We turned on the radio and danced to swing music. Not having these things helped me to keep my long childhood intact, and enjoy the 30's and 40's. It didn't leave me even after I married. I was still in a childlike way, (possibly because I married at eighteen).

In my early years, I learned to indulge in activities that were free. I attended the public library where I got all my questions answered with no complaints. I was happy. My wellness extended further with my participation in free games such as potsie, dodge ball, tag football, jacks, skelly, hide and seek, pool (on a neighbor's pool table), double dutch, bid whiz, checkers, chinese checkers, and most of all, handball (now called paddle ball).

I played handball during the day as well as into the evenings, no matter the weather, hot or very cold. My right hand became swollen from hitting the ball and sometimes one or two of my fingernails would scrape the ground. Broken and bloody, I stilled played on. The only activity that cost money was going to the movies. Every Saturday, we would see two full-length movies, a continuous action chapter clip, a cartoon, coming attractions, the news and we'd get a free dish as a gift. During those years, the price of a movie was ten cents for children.

In 1941 we were the first family to move into a new three-bedroom apartment in the Kings Borough Projects. The cost of rent was $4.00 a week, consistent with my parents' income. Ma said that some months had five weeks and the housing authority would get an extra four dollars in a five-week month. She felt that paying rent once a month was more appropriate to her pocketbook. We moved from a coal-water flat. It was approximately $15 Monthly. The New York City Housing Authority apartments always included gas, electric, hot water, and steam heat in the rent. I know Ma was really glad.

Also in 1941, the price of a subway fare was a nickel for adults and free for children under six. On the buses and trolleys adults still paid a nickel, but children under six were charged three cents (half fare). I was six forever.

Newspapers were two cents during the week and a nickel on Sunday. Post cards (existed then), were a penny and regular, sealed, first-class mail, was three cents. Precious gasoline was fifteen cents a gallon. No family member had a car except me. I became a driver at 20.

My childhood allowance was two cents from a deposit on a returned empty soda bottle and if I had two bottles to return, I felt rich. Ma also bought ice from the iceman for the icebox. I'm guessing that the ice was ten cents for a small block and fifteen cents for a larger one. I don't remember the price of milk, but it was home delivered and had heavy cream on the top. Usually, we kids enjoyed drinking this rich cream, never shaking it up. My parents cooked on a coal stove fueled by black coal. Our family room had a pop-belly stove.

Also, in 1941, schoolgirls wore a white middy blouse, navy blue skirt and a neat red scarf tied loosely around the neck of the blouse. The boys wore white shirts, a red tie, and navy-blue pants.

.

# Early Wellness

When going into wellness, please feel free to ask the question, *where in the heck do I begin?* The answer is to start at the beginning by simply cleaning out the body. Then slowly start weaning off bad foods and bad vices. Do this for thirty days. Use the same thirty days to slowly add on good organic food. After thirty days, you'll finally be the person you're supposed to be.

There is nothing like getting energy from the sun. There is nothing like fresh air deeply inhaled through the nostrils. There is nothing like carbon monoxide, toxins, poisons profoundly exhaled through the mouth. Take every opportunity to frequently practice deep breathing. Oxygen is our friend, and we use a lot of it when we breathe deeply. It is what helps the body move and be flexible. Oxygen feeds the mind before food feeds the stomach. It is the highest form of fuel for the body. The fuel that shapes our thoughts, our way of life, our way with words and our use of air. These sources give us better control over the choices we make. Let's give this air thing a try on the count of three 1...2...3...breath in, hold it for two seconds then, extend a long exhale. How do you feel? I know it feels like the best inhale/exhale of your life. Know that our oxygen has been restored to its ideal level when we do this. Continue this process three times a day or whenever possible. We must be aware of how vital air is to us. As we continue our journey, we're going to learn how choosing marvelous vegetables and fabulous fruits is crucial to a wellness lifestyle.

Early wellness is crucial for future wellness. A lost childhood is a shattered childhood, one which doesn't allow for a solid foundation. Where does one start in order to fit the pieces together, especially after reaching maturity? No one knows.

Early wellness is a chapter about growing up. Childhood is the foundation for adulthood. A well-built house has a foundation. A well-adjusted adult has a childhood, aka *'early wellness.'* Receiving wellness early is a must.

Wellness is a human instinct that adds value to the human race. Eating live foods offer great nutrition. Absorbing them promotes optimum cellular growth. Longevity is the goal, and it really is easy to pursue. Give yourself credit because you're the *matter of fact* that really matters most. You have the liberty to share your wellness with fellow brothers and sisters. What a life and what a delight!

Our parents and grandparents did not go to doctors except for an emergency. Whatever ails us, you can be sure they had a remedy to cure it. When you get a chance, ask an elder what they ate and drank to keep well. Allow him/her to inform you of their healing herbs and thank them for this needed knowledge (elder information is majestic). Seeing doctors younger than me makes me wonder if their healing plan will help them reach 92 (my age).

It won't hurt to ask your pharmacist about the side effects of the medication you were prescribed. The answer will be a surprise.

# Spiritual Wellness

**Question:** A kind way to show support for a fellow human being is_____ ?    (will answer later). It is not money.

I would like you to reflect on an occurrence that always happens. It is the union between a sperm, an egg, and a spirit. Nine months later, a bundle of joy arrives in the world. A brand-new innocent baby opens his/her arms, eyes, heart, and feelings to a spiritual awakening. Most babies are endowed with great health, nerves, glands, and a subconscious mind. It helps them to become familiar with mom and dad.

At first, parents have no idea how to handle this brand-new life experience. They're excited at the time and forget to ask the 64-thousand-dollar question, '*What can we parents do that would be beneficial to this brand-new family member?*' The answer to this question is simply composed of two little words - Grow up! Now the question becomes - how? A simple suggestion is this: One should never put energy into an unnatural force. It steers one in the wrong direction.

For example, innocent babies don't need parents who self-medicate. Young parents may think that this is the only solution to the pollution. It only urges one to eventually over medicate which eventually leads to stronger cravings. This is a process that happens when spirituality is left out of your life, especially if one is at a point of no return.
I repeat the two simple little words, GROW UP!

Parenthood is not easy, but it gets easier as you grow. Remember, God's gift to parents is a spiritual awakening. The responsibility of living a Godly life helps to build a strong foundation and merge wellness and spirituality as well as mental, moral, and physical standards.

The first notion of thinking is how to project better behavior which lifts us up where we belong. Snap to it. Don't waste a second. Allow yourself to quickly halt evil and immediately replace it with righteous behavior. The process is gradual and moves society closer to contentment. God wishes that we experience natural highs which promote spiritual elevation. Do this by breathing deeply through the nose, inhaling lots of oxygen, grasp it for a second, then release it. The inhalations open body passages which increase the amount of oxygen entering the lungs. Then, experience a long exhalation through the nose where carbon monoxide, toxins, poison and pain, will immediately be discharged.

The next step in assisting wellness is meditation. It allows relaxation to travel safely within the comfort zone of you and your sanity. It resolves anxiety and nervousness. It carries understanding and is the essence of satisfaction with no distractions.

Lastly, sincere prayer to the man above is a sincere connection to pursuing correction. It is the thing that deletes fear and apprehension. Consider the electric current connecting the need to continue the spiritual journey. Learn to manage a successful connection correction. All of the above equals peace and offers a spiritual life.

Another answer to the question is: Do everything you can to make life honest, straight forward, and easier for a fellow person. It's the best expression of spirituality.

The following are benefits toward a higher quality of living. Read it repeatedly until it sinks in. Sharing what you're hearing, (especially if its high-quality expressions), is spreading the connections that make the corrections. Are you picking up what I'm putting down?

One chooses happiness by making adjustments and beholding a lifestyle of wellness and peace. We have a statue of liberty, now, we need a statue of responsibility. Hurry. Connect to correct. Let us start heading towards connection to the correction. Give an example of how to be a solution to the pollution. This is happiness happening. This is spiritual wellness.

# Financial wellness

I earned capital from the following sources: employment, store owner, license real estate sale broker, homeowner, and an auto transporter. These were a few of the financial feats I pursued to achieve this wellness of finance.

I started working at age twelve, scrubbing my great Aunt Suzie's bathroom floors and a few other things she wanted done. She knew I needed a job, and I wanted to work, so I worked for her periodically.

Uncle Lem and Aunt Suzie were immaculate housekeepers. They had no children. At the nursing home where she was employed as a cook, there was an elderly female resident who needed cosmetic care. She needed body washing, hair combing and dressing as she was unable to do these things for herself. The nursing home preferred a neighborhood girl for the job, but since they couldn't find anyone, auntie was able to secure the job for me. With her recommendation, they gladly hired me. They paid me $5.00 a week plus carfare. I had to take two buses every day to get there. I delighted in having a regular job with a regular salary. It was a seven day a week job, most doable during my two-month summer vacation from school. This new job was my breakthrough. My financial wellness was born at that time. The door opened to my non-stop work history from 1945 to 2024.

In 1963, real estate broker Blaize, had a multiple dwelling for sale in Brownsville, Brooklyn. I met Mr. Blaize when he came to the retail store I shared with his friend, hat maker Robinson. My side of the store took orders for lady's wear; men's wear and children's wear. I called it the Vallura Shop and Mr. Robinson was the Allura Shop.

Broker Blaize was not a customer for us. He wanted his friend, Mr. Robinson, to purchase a building from him. I wasn't even an afterthought in this equation as women were not considered for such. After all, what could we do when an emergency occurred? Mr. Robinson declined the offer to purchase Mr. Blaize's multiple dwelling. Although I did not get an offer, nor any information and was excluded (even though I had a work history of eleven years with MTA and was a new proprietor of a retail store), Mr. Blaize did not want to even pursue a dry run with me, a woman. I didn't know it then, so I immediately became Ms. Buttinsky inquiring about the building. Since I made the first move, Mr. Blaize had no choice but to oblige. He politely suggested that I look at the property. Little did Mr. Blaize know, I had this house purchasing fever before owning the store, before MTA, before marrying Luther and before Ma complained about paying rent every week. My mind was made up. I wanted it even without seeing it. Mr. Blaize took me to see the multiple dwelling, and wouldn't you know it, it was the worst house on the block. Basically, I did not care about the negative condition of the property as long as it was a brick house, and it was. I had no doubt that the positive reasons for purchasing such a property would outweigh the negatives. Anyway, I reasoned, I needed a place to put my beat-up car and since it was a semi-detached house, I'd have a parking space. Thank God the first floor was occupied with tenants, otherwise it would have been worst (if possible).

I agreed to purchase it, but I had no money. I immediately stipulated that the seller wave the down-payment of $1,000 until after I obtained the mortgage and collected the rent. They were very happy to do this, so it was agreed to without hesitation. After all, why lose a customer especially since the house was dilapidated and no one else wanted it. I was the only one who saw the vision for this house as a place to live and pay rent to myself. Also, the vision of being a homeowner and building equity was good even though at thirty years of age,

I didn't clearly understand such a term as equity. I did know that procuring real estate enabled me to see where my money was invested and to monitor it. Like I previously said, I, and only one other person saw the vision: my godmother's husband Pop Colbert. Other than him, the whole world saw so many negative things about a woman becoming a buyer of a building. This gave me an education no school could ever give me, and I appreciated it.

## "We've Come This Far By Faith"

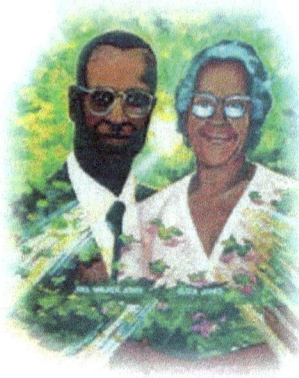

**Joel Walker Jones "Poppy"**

(1884-1957)

**Eliza Brown Jones "Liza"**

(1890-1961)

Joseph Connolly Jones "Toots"

Fred Lee Jones

George Edward Jones

Blanche Orethea Jones Green Smith "Sis"

Gladys Patilda Jones McCabe "Date"

Melford David Jones "Brot"

Thomas Bernard Jones "Tom"

Dorothy Vernice Jones Glaude "Dot"

Jerome Walker Jones, Sr. "Jerry"

# Family Wellness

Family. The word alone is so heartfelt.

I was five years old when the love of my life, Grandma Mattie, was admitted to the hospital diagnosed with a nervous breakdown. She never returned home. Grandma was in her late fifties. Seventeen years later, when I was twenty-two, Grandpa Nat died in his mid-seventies. He had cancer of the throat. Ma died at the age of sixty-five, leaving most of her pension untouched. She retired because she was ill. Ma was a heavy smoker, and I believe her lungs collapsed.

Both of my sisters were skinny before puberty. After puberty (age 13), weight zoomed onto their bodies and continued to escalate. They were not active people, in fact, they were the absolute opposite. Sister Margaret never went anywhere, which was unusual for a New York girl. She stayed home because she did not want to be teased about being short (4' 9"). Margaret made home a safe haven that she never left. Ma was so glad to condone Margaret's home ship (this added another plus to her first-born daughter). In reality, it created more stress for Margaret and initiated a sickness called asthma. My sister suffered a lot throughout her 49 years of living. I remember her saying, *"I thought I was going to die after my last attack."* It was actually a prayer for relief, and it was answered. She made her transition in January 1980 at the age of forty-nine.

Sister Jackie went on a retreat to a fat farm for two weeks. I remember the small amount of weight she lost. The weight just came right back as soon as she returned home. Jackie never went back again. Everything she tried was more discouraging than encouraging.

Both Margaret and Jackie both had uneventful lifestyles. They were the last two people who needed to live together. This led them right back to where they were, overweight without a clue. They knew that they were good girls and that's all that ultimately mattered to them. Even after Margaret died in January 1980, Sister Jackie continued her behavior. Margaret's death did not compel her to live any differently. She did visit Spain, as well as take a few college courses. It was like two drops in a great big bucket.

Sister Jackie was admitted to the hospital in 1982 (age 38) weighing 333 lbs. She also suffered cardiac arrest. The doctors brought her back but didn't give any hope of her surviving too much longer. Her medical history read: heart failure, kidney failure, obesity, high blood pressure, pneumonia, fluid retention and eventually she became a dialysis patient. With my assistance and my wellness ideas (even back then), I added seven years to her life. At the end of the seven years, she was tired of dialysis and decided not to continue. She died April 30, 1989.

The deaths of my parents were sad and, I thought, premature, because they only made it to 65 years of age. The deaths of my sisters were also premature, but more shocking and painful. Neither of them reached the age of ma, grandma, grandpa, or my father. They died too young.

They had an easy life, living a limited lifestyle which caused them to experience the shortest lifetime in the immediate family. Their style of living left wellness out of their lives and I often wondered why they did everything in their power to leave it out. A rhetorical question, but Margaret and Jackie unequivocally reinforced my wellness lifestyle. Seeing both my sisters' style of living caused me to seek a passionate healing structure. They're why I walk the path of wellness today and every day with vows to be well (especially when thoughts of my sisters arise, which happens frequently). I go deep into thinking and knowing, that I would protect the life God gave me. My health and I are close knit, vigorously doing the work to stay attuned. I utilize fortitude, buoyancy, flexibility, resilience, and willpower for wellness. All strength from God the Almighty to whom I pay homage.

Is listening to your parent's family wellness? My answer is yes and no. Why both answers—because most people become parents prior to arriving at the required maturity to do the job properly. Within many families, the subject isn't addressed (my family missed this point also). Yes, we should listen to our parents because they did the best they could while raising us. We simply do not recognize the main reason for kinfolk as well as not being able to put it into plain words. Most of us become parents or family leaders before we are equipped to do the job. So, let's face the issue now. Family meetings build family wisdom. Family members attending family meetings can express the words that decipher their objectives. The following is my suggested lingo: Compromise, conciliate, confront, give a little, take a little, negotiate.

Another issue is: accomplishing healthy family relations and good family wisdom through one word: **"RESPECT."** Young children want their parents to respect each other. Nothing else will satisfy them. Please know RESPECT between people who birth a family is a great gift for all involved. Otherwise, our children feel that they are the cause of family disagreements. Children blame themselves for the grueling family arguments between mom, dad, and other family members. These issues, endowed with evil, destroy family relationships. Some parents try to solve their troubles with favoritism or by giving games and other playthings, etc. to replace the disrespect. It takes patience to achieve family esteem which only mature humans can pull off. To continue in this obstinate way, wipes out family living (mother and father with children). Like most things today however, respect seems to be labeled old-fashioned. I hope you and others will pray for this 'old fashioned' virtue to come back.

Parenting classes have never been enforced in high schools, nor has it been added to college curricula. A strong family foundation is the standard tool. Having monthly meetings is a smart tool to help air family differences. Not doing so is a family slip-up. Many families make the same mistake. Even my family never saw the need for family dialogue. Whatever mother said was final. Some of it must have been incorrect since my only two sisters never dated and never got married. They accepted mother's decisions. She was always right as far as they knew. Since father wasn't around, mother made the decisions, and they were concrete. I, on the other hand, saw that a correction was needed. They didn't see it. Please utilize family dialogue as a simple solution to SOAR toward family wellness.

Are we ready to make this adjustment to correct the ongoing family struggle? Are we ready to stop blocking family wellness and let healing happen? Are we ready to keep family hope alive? I'm sure you'll answer all of the above with a big YES!

# Disease Prevention Wellness Extension Connections

Unlock the blocks you hold against WELLNESS and employ the following caring list to immediately dismiss disease. I explain this as: Disease Prevention Wellness Extension Connections.

## The Well Life Help (List)

1. Acupuncture
2. Colon Cleansing
3. Catalyst Altered Water (CAW),
4. Movements of Dance (Dr. Day's Video *'Cancer Doesn't Scare Me'* is a video in my library)
5. The Farmers' Market
6. Food Co-ops
7. Gyms
8. Neighborhood health coaches
9. Holistic Teams
10 Saunas and steam rooms

11 Vegetable juices

12 Yoga

Add your own pathway gems to this health connection/correction list.

The above DPWEC's are huge. Get excited about its magnitude. Feel the wellness blossoming and permit it to continue. Get it all. Leap into spring, summer, winter, and fall. My thoughts are to simply use your health as a target for success. Hurry, it is an expedition, so make it your healing mission. Your regenerated organs will thank you and my thanks will be with you as well. GOD will genuinely thank you for keeping His temple in an A-OK condition.

More healing tips and ideas are in my first book, *'I'M A WELLNESS WITNESS,'* published in November 2018. In it, you'll find healthy rhymes, a chapter (called MOTHER WIT), with clever language that brings witty thoughts to mind. Hurry, get your copy from Barnes & Nobles or Amazon.

Don't miss an opportunity to read about our *real* medicine - organic fruits and vegetables. It's the food that builds a strong immune system.

Hear ye! There are 24-hour emergency clinics in every city for people who are non-wholistic. There are no emergency clinics for wholistic patients, this is unfair. I believe a solution to this can be solved with our churches. The first church that takes on this responsibility will go down in history. Wholistic patients will be more than glad to make a donation for this service of fresh vegetable and fruit juices. We need to connect to correct this error. Our civil rights leaders always had plenty of fresh fruits and vegetables. (very little fast-food). Think about how this contributed to their success in winning Black civil rights. Think again. Six hundred-pound humans were never heard of in their time. There was no such being. Eating healthy fresh meats, vegetables and fruits gave them the strength to fight for civil rights.

Wellness connections or wellness pathways are pleasant introductions within both of my books. I made an adjustment and took the privileged to portray: Disease Prevention, Wellness Extension Connection to Correction.

This tongue twister will hopefully steer society toward becoming wellness leaders. This way, fresh, new, innovative people will expand on ideas to foster good health. These wellness leaders will spread glowing healing stories with enough excitement to light a fuse. This lighted fuse will ignite society to finally choose fitting and feasible lifestyles of strength, not weakness. In this book, there is special knowledge on making good health a cinch and poor health nothing to clinch. Open your heart to see the need for the corrections that lead to a good health seed. Revitalize and *'Let there be Wellness'* work as a superior guide to enjoy a super healthy life.

# Fashion Wellness

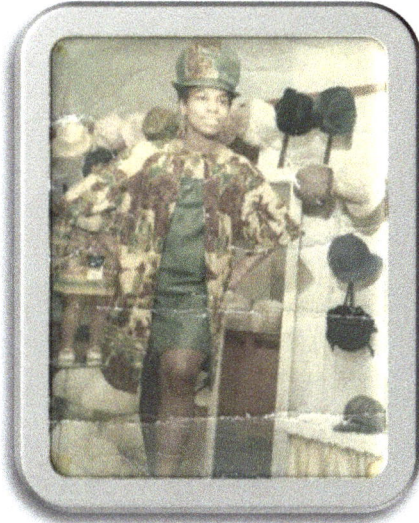

**June Terry creations. Etta Dixon - Model**

Ms. June Terry has been a New Yorker since 1947. She is the mother of six children: one boy, three girls and a set of twin girls. She's a grandmother of four and a great-grandmother of two.

Terry graduated from the Fashion Institute of Technology (FIT). Later, she received the award for excellence in black theatre. She has a background of pattern making and costume designing for women and she knows how to dress women.

She went to Ghana in October of 2003 and lived there for five years. She really fused with the culture of Africa, especially with what they wore. She noticed first that their clothes were comfortable. When she came back to America, she brought this exciting fact back with her.

I remember in the 60's, African Americans were starred for dashikis. They were filled with color, combined with brightness and comfort.

Thank you, June! Please remember Ms. Terry's motto: Wear comfortable clothes!

# Tips for Self-care

### Dance

You can never go wrong.

### Wash the Eyes

Dry eye is common, particularly in older adults. Tears provide lubrication, reduce the risk of eye infection, and wash away foreign debris.

### Open Pill Bottles

If you have a condition like arthritis, you may need pill bottles that are easier to open than the standard child proof containers that come with most medications.

### Wash the Ears

When excess earwax accumulates in the ear canal, it can harden. Earwax buildup is more common among older adults because the consistency of earwax changes with age. Carefully wipe the insides of your ears at home. Some seniors may need the help of a medical professional for a thorough cleaning.

**Good oral hygiene is critical for your health.** Read about the top three electric toothbrushes for older adults.

Kids toothbrushes are more comfortable for seniors.

# PORTRAITS
## Of life

*(Most are very old. Remember, I'm 92 years young!)*

My High School graduation

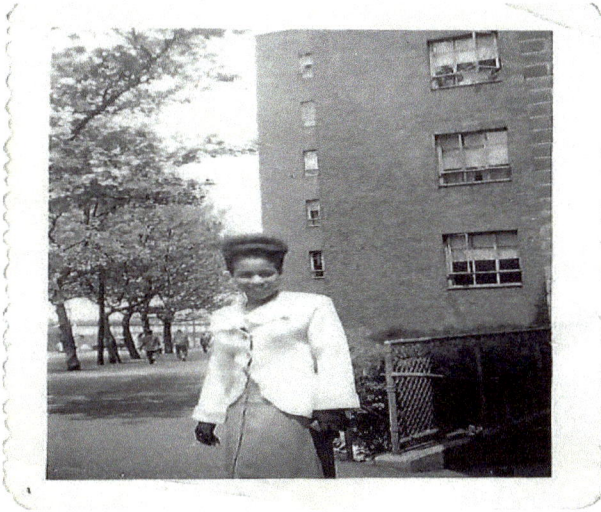

Showing off my first car: A Lincoln Continental

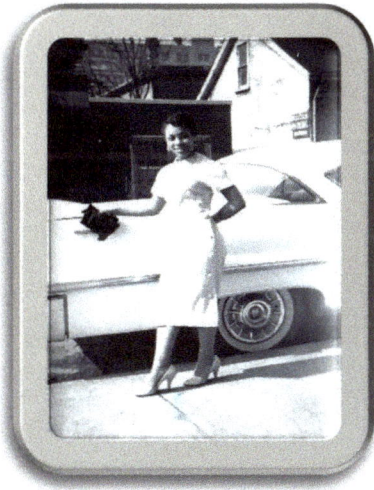

Relaxing at a resort

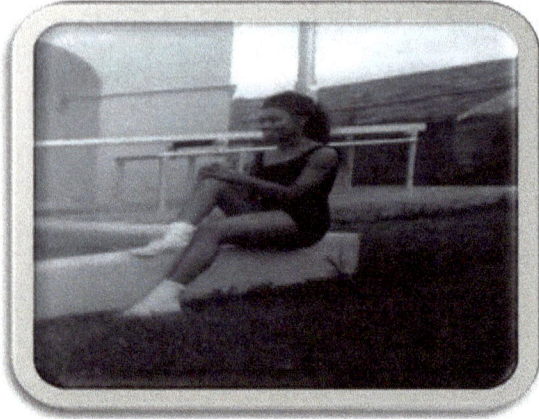

In front of my store

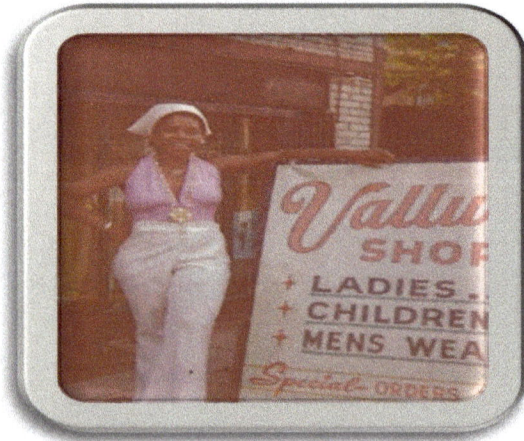

Getting ready for a drive

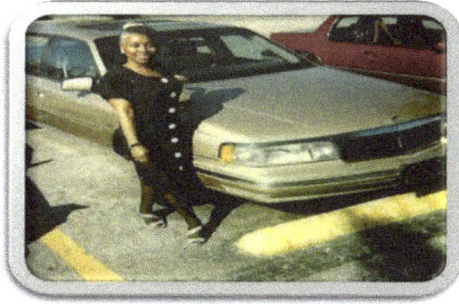

Having fun at the King Spa in NJ

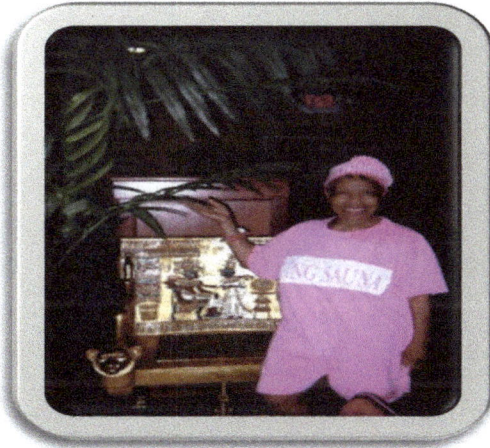

Getting ready to write my next book

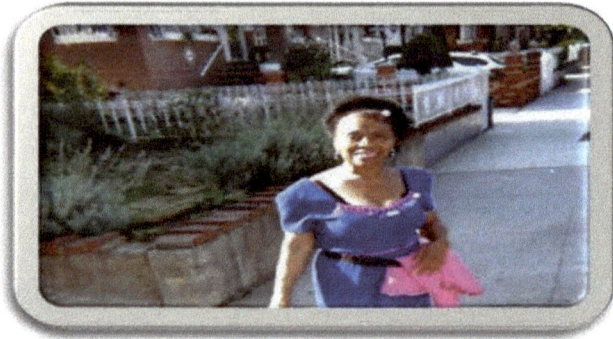

Photoshoot for my first book

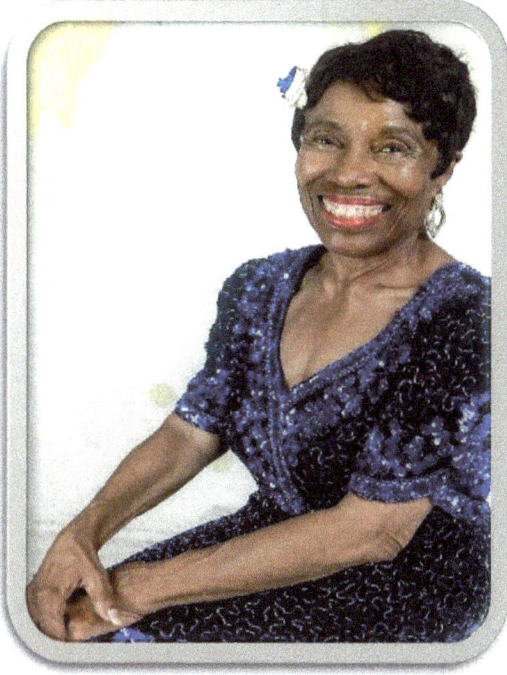

# FAMILY & FRIENDS

My Mom getting ready to say her piece

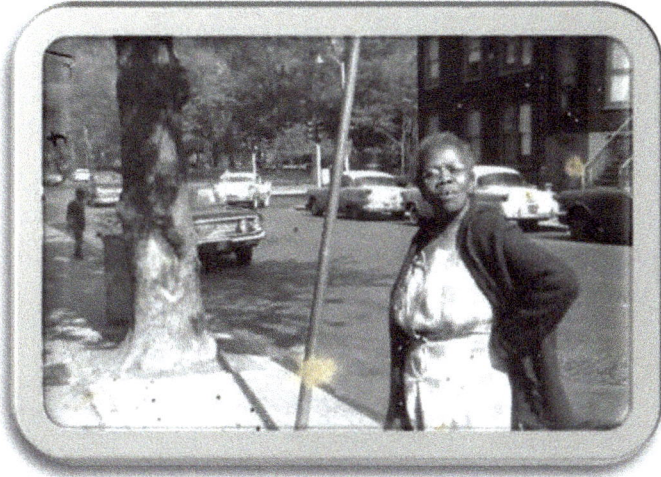

My sister Jackie – age 8

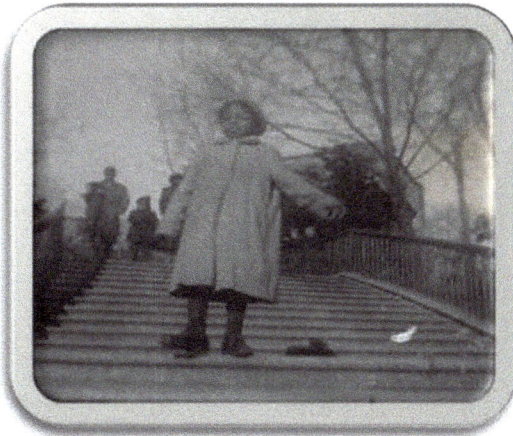

# My Wedding August 9, 1952

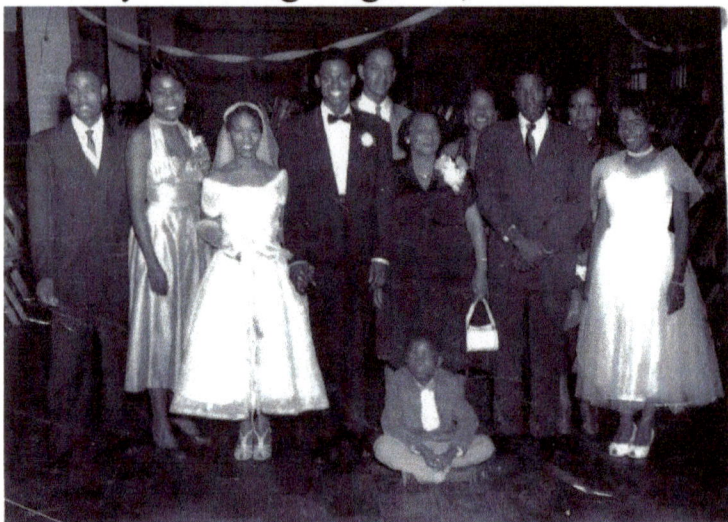

# My sister-in-law's wedding

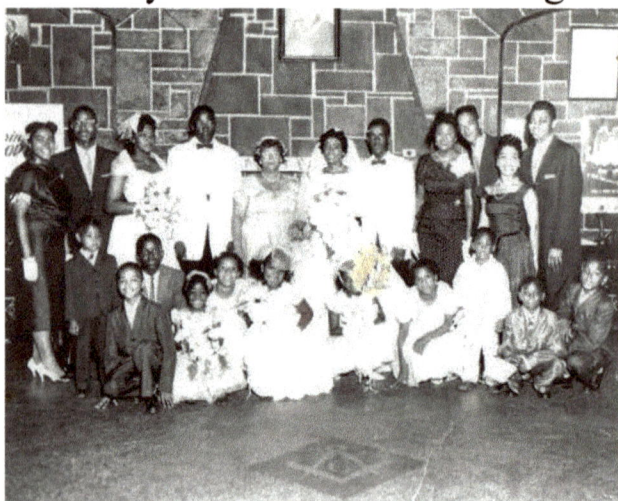

Together with friends

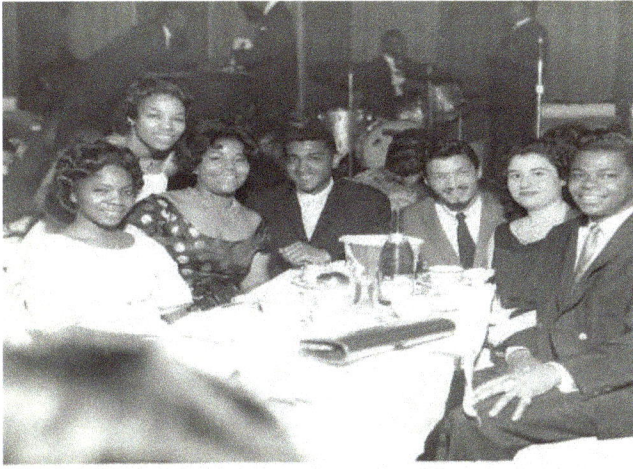

Husband Luther (middle) enjoying his buddies

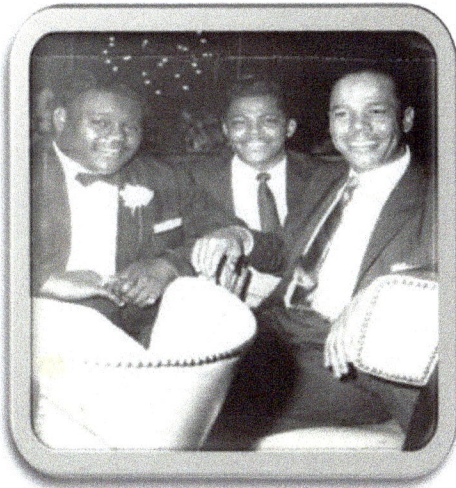

Husband Luther playing tennis. Enjoying a
fun day in the sun

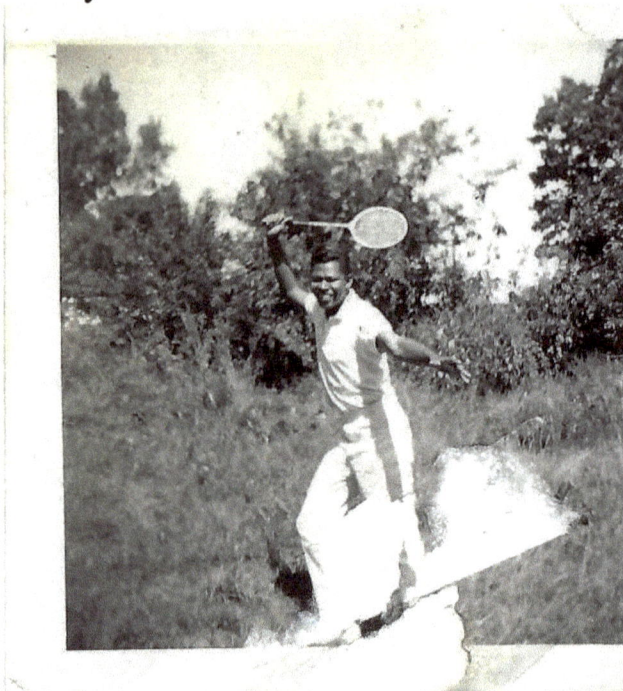

# Celebrities I've Met

Award day for Etta!

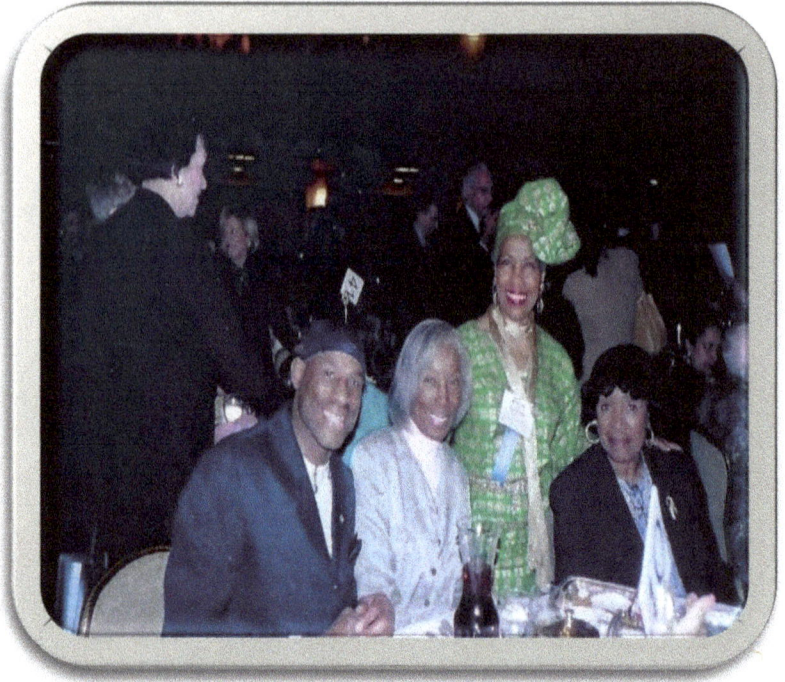

Brookdale hospital Top Volunteer!

## Danny Glover

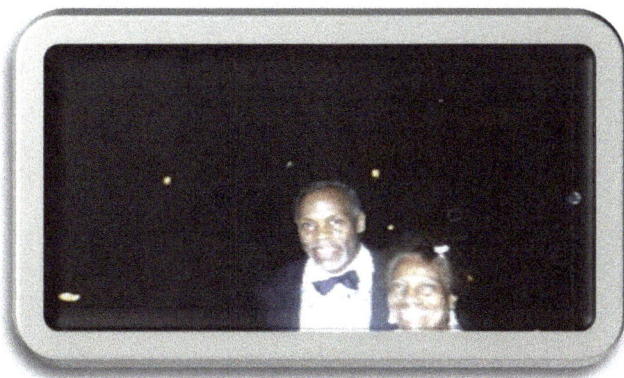

## Chuck Jackson

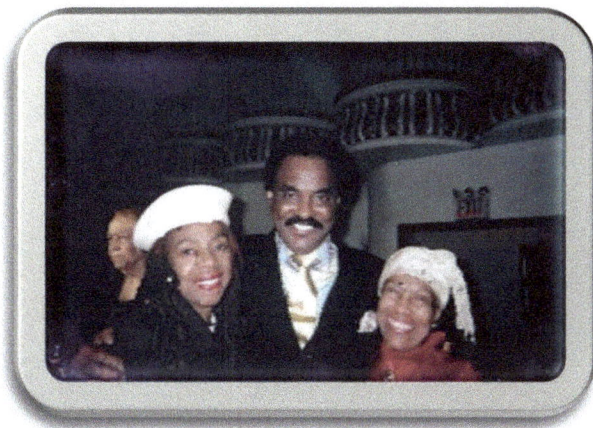

## Queen Afua

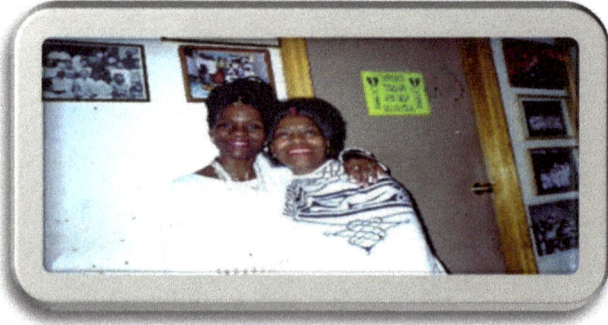

## David Dinkins

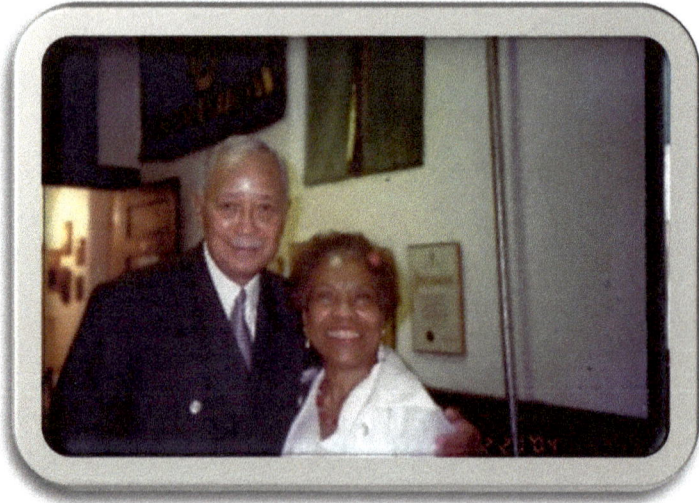

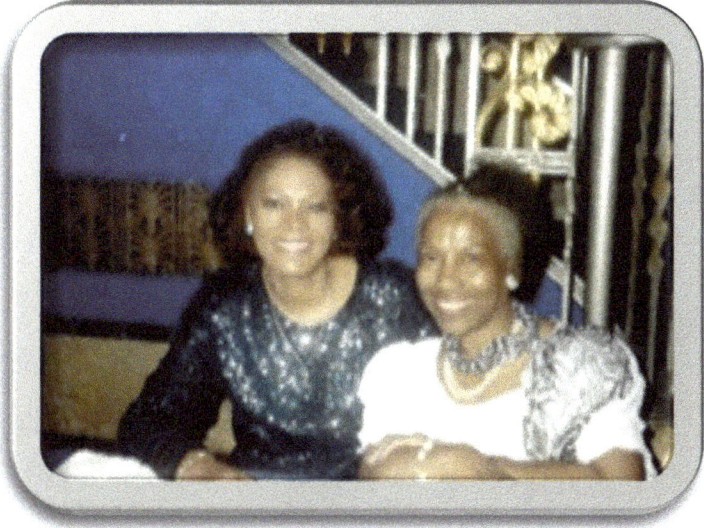

*Dionne Warwick*

# About the Author

Miss Etta Dixon is a rare nonagenarian as she's in optimal health! She's a living testament to the messages in both of her books. *I'm a Wellness Witness* and *Let there be Wellness (Don't Block It!)*.

On the following pages, keep a journal of your path to wellness. I'm rooting for you!

Etta Dixon

www.ingramcontent.com/pod-product-compliance
Lightning Source LLC
Chambersburg PA
CBHW040141270326
41928CB00022B/3284